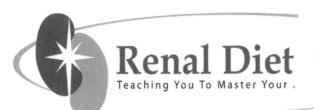

D1627116

Eating A Pre-Dialysis Kidney Diet — Sodium, Potassium, Phosphorus, and Fluids

Book 2

Mathea Ford, RD/LD

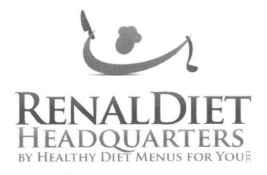

RENALDIET HEADQUARTERS
BY HEALTHY DIET MENUS FOR YOU

Purpose and Introduction

What I have found through the emails and requests of my readers is that it is difficult to find information about a pre-dialysis kidney diet that is actionable. I want you to know that is what I intend to provide in all my book. You can take these recipes from our website and information to create meals that you and your family will enjoy and they all fit a stage 2 – 5 kidney disease patient.

I wrote this book with you in mind: the person with kidney problems who does not know where to start or can't seem to get the answers that you need from other sources. This book will provide information that is applicable to a predialysis kidney disease diet.

Who am I? I am a registered dietitian in the USA who has been working with kidney patients for my entire 15 + years of experience. Find all my books on Amazon on my author page: http://www.amazon.com/Mathea-Ford/e/Boo8E1E7IS/

My goals are simple – to give some answers and to create an understanding of what is typical. In this series of 12 books, I will take you through the different parts of being a person with pre-dialysis kidney disease. It will not necessarily be what happens in your case, as everyone is an individual. I may simplify things in an effort to write them so that I feel you can learn the most from the information. This may mean that I don't say the exact things that your doctor would say. If you don't understand, please ask your doctor.

I want you to know, I am not a medical doctor and I am not aware of your particular condition. Information in this book is current as of publication, but may or may not have changed. This book is not meant to substitute for medical treatment for you, your friends, your caregivers, or your family members. You should not base treatment decisions solely on what is contained in this book. Develop your treatment plan with your doctors, nurses and the other medical professionals on your team. I recommend that you double-check any information with your medical team to verify if it applies to you.

In other words, I am not responsible for your medical care. I am providing this book for information and entertainment purposes, not medical diagnoses. Please consult with your doctor about any questions that you have about your particular case.

If you would be interested in getting more information about specifics related to sodium amounts in certain foods, meal planning sheets, and low sodium spices and flavoring tips, please sign up for the email list at:

Go to: http://www.renaldiethq.com/book2files/

It's a supplement to the book, this book is complete. But it will add to your knowledge! We also share our latest information with you so you are always informed.

TABLE OF CONTENTS

General Information about Micronutrients and Your Diet

You need micronutrients (sodium, potassium, and phosphorus) in your diet the same way that you need macronutrients (carbohydrates, fats, and protein). They do not contribute calories to your daily intake, but can affect your kidneys and other organs in a significant way. They add flavor to foods as well as nutritional value. For someone with kidney disease, they can be a problem unless you understand what is happening with your condition and what amounts you can and cannot eat.

In this section, I will discuss the main micronutrients that are important to a kidney diet: Sodium, Potassium, and Phosphorus.

Salt or Sodium – What Does It Matter?

Salt and sodium are abundant in our food supply, and are used mainly to preserve and add flavor to foods. So a product that is canned will have more sodium than a fresh or frozen product because of the way that product is processed. Your body needs less than 1,000 milligrams per day to do normal biological functions, but the normal American diet contains about 5,000 mg.

Salt is a mineral that is a combination of two elements – sodium and chloride. So, sodium can be part of many different chemical combinations – MSG for example is mono – sodium – glutamate. When you read a label, look in the ingredients panel for items that use the word sodium in the name. In other words, sodium content listed on the label does not just come from salt – it comes from many items. Either way, the number on the nutrition label listed under sodium is the one you should be concerned with. When reading recipes and ingredients, you can estimate if it will have a lot of sodium by reading the names. Many products contain high amounts of sodium – table salt, soy sauce, and teriyaki sauce for example. Canned foods, snack foods, and most processed meats also contain large amounts of salt.

SODIUM CAN BE HARMFUL BECAUSE OF THE EFFECT ON BLOOD PRESSURE

When you eat a lot of sodium, it can be harmful because it can cause your body to retain fluid. When you have CKD (Chronic Kidney Disease), you want to be sure not to let too much fluid build up in your blood and tissues. That can raise your blood pressure and put more strain on your heart and kidneys. Studies have shown that sodium is handled differently in the kidneys by persons with chronic kidney disease.

The recommendation from the US Government is that generally healthy persons should aim to consume less than 2,400 mg of sodium per day. (That is one teaspoon of table salt). If you have high blood pressure or kidney disease, you should aim for no more than 1,500 mg per day.

What happens when your blood pressure is high? The increase in your blood pressure damages the blood vessels in your kidneys. They are susceptible because they are small and sensitive to many changes in your body. When you have an elevation in your blood pressure, it can scar the small capillaries (blood vessels) in your kidneys and cause them to be destroyed. That reduces the overall filtering capacity of your kidneys. Did your doctor tell you that you have 20% of your kidney function left? Basically, about 80% of your small capillaries are damaged at that point. When your blood pressure is increased over 130 mm Hg systolic (top) number, you have double the risk of heart attack and stroke. Heart disease is the number one cause of death amongst people with kidney disease. I don't mean to scare you but this is serious.

Using other seasonings can help with lowering your sodium intake. A salt free seasoning mix or Tabasco sauce can spice up the flavor without adding additional sodium. Lemon juice can add a lot to flavor a dish without adding salt. Avoid using the "salt substitutes" that are made with potassium chloride. These are items such as Nu-Salt and AlsoSalt that increase your potassium intake which is another mineral you should be watching on a kidney diet.

Preparing foods from scratch, and using recipes, are the best ways to decrease your intake of sodium because the majority of the salt in our diet is from manufacturers adding salt to foods. So, if you are making the meal, you control how much sodium or salt is put in the food. Recipes need some salt, but many times recipes can be revised to reduce the amount of sodium without losing taste.

You will also need to relearn the way food tastes so you can use less salt in your food. It can take a few weeks, but your taste buds will adjust. You will be experiencing the "real" flavor of food, not the salt.

Some options for lower sodium foods are:

> Salt-free herb seasonings
> Low sodium canned foods
> Frozen vegetables without sauce
> Fresh, cooked meats
> Plain rice without sauce
> Plain noodles without sauce
> Fresh vegetables without sauce
> Homemade soup with fresh ingredients
> Reduced sodium tomato paste
> Unsalted pretzels
> Unsalted popcorn

Keys to Reducing Sodium in Your Diet

1. Don't add salt to your food in cooking or at the table
2. Read labels and choose foods with 300 mg sodium or less per serving
3. Reduce your intake of the following foods:

   a. Soy Sauce
   b. Fast Food Items
   c. Cured or processed meats and cheeses
   d. Salted Snack Foods
   e. Vegetables that are canned or processed with salt

When you are concerned and trying to reduce the overall sodium in your diet, you can take multiple steps to lower the intake of sodium.

STEPS TO TAKE TO LOWER THE SODIUM IN YOUR DIET:
Use recipes that involve less salt or reduce the amount of salt you put into them.
Limit your use of processed foods like microwave meals and canned foods.
Read the labels on seasoning packets for added salts
Eat less hard cheeses, pickles, olives, hot dogs and other deli meats that are not reduced sodium
Avoid the use of salt substitutes with potassium instead of sodium – you will need to limit your intake of potassium as well during kidney disease. You can use Mrs. Dash or other salt-free blend that does not use potassium.
Read the labels on over the counter medications – many contain added sodium for flavor.

Use a variety of herbs and spices to flavor your food. Rub them together between your hands to release a little more flavor. If you are using dried herbs instead of fresh, use about 25-50% less than called for.

Use vinegar and lemon juice to flavor your foods. I love adding a little butter and lemon juice to my rice to add flavor without added salt.

You don't need to add salt to water when boiling pasta or rice.

Top 4 Ways To Reduce Sodium In Your Diet

By now, you probably realize that sodium restriction is an important part of a renal diet. Eating a lower sodium diet, and watching where your sodium comes from helps slow the progression of your kidney disease. Which is what you would like to do, right?

You probably already know that the amount of sodium you should eat in a day is the equivalent of about 1 teaspoon. Also known as approximately 2400 mg per day. As a person on a renal diet, your aim should be slightly lower than that – in the 1500 mg per day range.

Let's talk about ways you can reduce the sodium in your diet.

Cook at home more often. Bottom line - you have complete control over the amount of sodium that goes into your meal when you're cooking at home and have a choice of what you put into the meal. Choosing not to add the extra salt, or rinsing your canned vegetables before you put them into the recipe, or using frozen vegetables - all contribute to a lower sodium meal.

Eat more whole food snacks. No, I'm not talking about going to the Whole Foods Market and buying snacks. But I am talking about eating less processed snacks. Eating an apple for a snack is a low potassium low phosphorous choice. If you were to eat applesauce, you would not get as much fiber and you would possibly get a little more sodium in your snack. When I say whole food, I'm referring to the less processed version of a meal or snack. Something that is closer to what it would be found like in nature.

Speaking of whole food snacks, eating fruits and vegetables as part of both your meals and snacks every time lowers your sodium and increases the fiber that you intake. Fresh fruits in season can be reasonably priced. And if you don't like the fresh fruit in season you can grab a bag of the frozen fruits and snack on those. A bowl of strawberries with some artificial sweetener or sugar can be a great snack. Frozen and fresh vegetables have the least amount of sodium. When compared to the canned vegetable, the sodium in a fresh or frozen vegetable is negligible. Choose fresh vegetables when they're in season, and the rest of the year eat the frozen version. Either way, take up half your plate with fruits and vegetables and you'll be lower in sodium and much healthier.

Cut back on condiments. You may not realize it but ketchup has a lot of sodium in it. I'm aware that on a renal diet you're not necessarily going to be eating a lot of ketchup or tomatoes, but almost every condiment is processed and has added sodium. Barbecue sauce, mustard, and salad dressings all are higher in sodium. For salad dressing as an example, you could use oil and vinegar instead of a process salad dressing and that would decrease the amount of sodium that you had in that salad.

I know it's hard to reduce the amount of sodium that you have in your diet especially when you eat out a lot or you eat a lot of processed foods. But the awareness that you need to follow a renal diet should help you to make this positive choices and take some of the steps that are going to be vital to reducing your sodium intake, and therefore improving your kidney function.

SALT FREE BREAD RECIPE

Ingredients

2 cups warm water

3 tablespoons vegetable oil

3 tablespoons sugar

2 (1/4 ounce) package fast rising yeast

5 -6 cups flour

Directions

Put water in large bowl. Add oil and sugar, then yeast. Mix in a little flour and let stand a few minutes until bubbles start to form. Stir in flour (may use mixer) until thick batter. Then add flour slowly until dough starts to come from sides of bowl.

Turn onto floured surface, round into ball. Cover with bowl. Let stand 10 minutes. Knead, adding flour if necessary so it isn't sticky. Dough should feel smooth and soft.

Put into well oiled bowl. Turn so it is covered with oil. Cover with towel. Should double in size in about half hour or a little more. Punch down and divide into 2 loaves.

Put into well oiled or sprayed 9 5/8 x 5 1/2 x 2 3/4 inch pans. Oil tops, let rise until doubled in size. Set in oven. Turn heat to 350 degrees. Bake about an hour or until loaves are brown on top and pull away from sides of pan. Put on rack to cool. Makes excellent toast. If cut into 16 slices, 97 calories per slice.

Tips For Reading Your Food Labels

The US government regulates the terminology that can be used on a food's label. Some terms and their meanings can help you understand what you are looking for without having to turn the product around and read the label.

Sodium Free – Very little sodium in each serving

Very Low Sodium – 35 milligrams of sodium or less in each serving

Low Sodium – 140 mg of sodium or less in each serving

Reduced Sodium – Sodium has been lowered by 25% from the "regular" product. If it were potato chips – the new product that states reduced sodium would have 25% less sodium in each serving than the regular potato chips

Light in Sodium – Sodium has been lowered by at least 50% (similar to the above situation for reduced sodium)

Nutrition Label Reading For Sodium Content

Each food label is required to show the amount of sodium per serving. As I said before, if you have a product that is 140 mg of sodium or less, you can consider that a low sodium product and include it in your diet.

On the other hand, if a product contains 300 mg or more of sodium per serving, that amount is too high for you to consume.

Look at labels for the following statements that indicate it is a good choice for sodium reduced diets: Sodium Free, Salt Free, Very Low Sodium, Low Sodium, Reduced or Less Sodium, Light in Sodium, No salt added, Unsalted, Lightly Salted.

Choose cereals that contain less than 280 mg of sodium per serving and frozen meals (TV Dinners) that contain less than

600 mg per serving (Because it contains multiple courses of the meal, instead of just one item). **Remember to try to stick to 1,500 mg per day of sodium**.

HOW DO I FIND LOW SODIUM FOODS?

When you're looking for low sodium foods, reading labels is one of the most important things that you can do. Comparing the exact same product may show that one pasta sauce has 80 mg of sodium and another pasta sauce has 400 mg per serving. Make sure the serving size is the same and choose wisely. An example might be: the one with 400 mg of sodium might be a 1/4 cup serving, and the one with 80 mg might be ½ cup serving – so it's a better choice.

Eat more fruits and vegetables, especially those that are frozen or fresh. Canned fruits and vegetables can be higher in sodium, so choosing a frozen product may give you a fresher meal and reduce sodium altogether. Eat fruits that are in season that match your potassium requirement. Try to mix in extra vegetables when making soups and casseroles to make them tastier and more filling.

Speaking of mixing extra vegetables into soups and casseroles, **it's very important that you prepare more meals from scratch at home**. No matter how you slice it, you really need to eat those foods that are not coming from boxes or frozen convenience foods, but something that you made that you can control the amount of sodium per serving.

Finally, look at the portion size of foods that you're eating. You may find a pasta sauce with only 80 mg but determined that the serving size is only 1 tablespoon. You're definitely going to eat more pasta sauce than that. So when you're comparing make sure that you're aware of how much are actually going to eat of the product.

DOES THE DASH DIET CONTAIN THE RIGHT ITEMS FOR ME TO EAT?

The DASH Diet (Dietary Approaches To Stopping Hypertension) is a recommended diet for some people with mild kidney damage. If you have stage 1 or 2 kidney disease, it might be the right diet for you and you should consider looking at more ways to increase your intake of whole vegetables and fruits.

But the DASH diet contains a higher protein, potassium, and phosphorus content than is recommended for patients with CKD Stages 3-5.

The amount of protein in the DASH diet is approximately 1.4 gm/kg/day. It is considered optimal for persons with stage 3 or 4 kidney failure to take in only about .8 gm/kg/day of protein. More than that is difficult for your kidneys to process and can cause problems for your entire body. It is imperative that you watch protein, potassium, phosphorus and sodium in stages 3-4.

POTASSIUM – ANOTHER MINERAL YOU MIGHT NEED TO COUNT!

Keeping your potassium levels in check is an important part of your diet as you progress in stages through kidney disease. Early on, in stages 1 and 2, you could eat a higher amount of potassium and not be as concerned because your kidneys could still handle it. They could remove the potassium and not let it build up in your blood.

> If Your Serum (blood) Potassium is 5.0 mEq/L or higher, you should restrict your potassium intake.
>
> Hyperkalemia (high blood potassium) is usually not seen until CKD is advanced, but may be seen at higher eGFR's (lower stages) in people with diabetes and CKD.

But in stages 3 – 5, you will possibly need to limit the amount that you take in. Now, watching how much you eat and how your body responds, will be the key to slowing the progression of kidney disease.

You probably already know how potassium can affect your kidneys. I think your key question should be – do I need to reduce my intake of potassium? Potassium works to keep muscles pumping, and one of the largest muscles in your body is your heart. You don't want the blood levels too high or too low. Damaged kidneys can allow the potassium to build up in the blood instead of being removed – and that can cause heart problems.

Your doctor will tell you if you need to lower potassium, and if you do – it's usually in the 2-3 gm per day range.

IF YOU NEED TO LOWER POTASSIUM...

If your physician has instructed you to eat less potassium, you need to follow their instructions. But if they have not given you any indication about eating more or less potassium, use the guideline in the box – if your labs show that your serum potassium is 5.0 mEq/L or higher, start limiting your potassium.

If you don't know your lab numbers – call your doctor's office and get a copy right now. They will give them to you. And if they have not done a serum potassium – ask them to order it and go get it done. You need to know!

Look at your food labels as well – in the ingredients section – for the words potassium. That will be a huge indication of the need to restrict that food or not. Ingredients are required to be listed in the order of the amount (by weight) in the food. The first ingredient is the item that the product has the most of.

I am also going to get into the foods to eat and not eat, but for a moment I want to remind you that you can "leach" vegetables to make them lower in potassium. When you leach vegetables, you go through a process of slicing and soaking that enables the potassium to be released from the vegetable.

LEACHING, EXPLAINED...

Some foods that you really want to eat are high potassium foods. And it's hard to not be able to eat them because they are a potassium rich foods. You can do several things to lower the amount of potassium and help you in your quest to achieve a low potassium diet. Learning how to leach vegetables to reduce the amount of potassium is a basic skill that is very important to you when cooking for a renal diet. You will need more potassium restriction as your kidney failure worsens, and while on dialysis. So, being able to still eat some of the high potassium foods by leaching vegetables will enable you to continue to have some variety in your diet.

What is leaching? Leaching is the process of removing potassium out of vegetables by soaking and other means so that the vegetable releases some of it's potassium instead of ingesting it. Learning how to leach vegetables is a valuable practice for people on a kidney diet to allow for continued variety of foods. Leaching reduces the amount of potassium in vegetables to 25-50% of the original value. The longer you soak them, the warmer the water, and the smaller the pieces make the difference in how much potassium is removed.

NOW, LET'S GET STARTED LEARNING HOW TO LEACH VEGETABLES

High potassium foods need to be prepped for eating by leaching the potassium out of them. This usually takes about 2-4 hours.

Potatoes, sweet potatoes, carrots, beets, and rutabagas require the following process:

Prepare a pot with cold water that is large enough to hold the amount of vegetable you are preparing.

Peel the vegetable and slice it about 1/8th inch thick (or as thin as you can), place the slices in the cold water to prevent them from turning brown

Once you have peeled all the vegetables, empty the pot, and rinse the vegetables in warm water. Then fill the pot back up - using about 10 times the amount of water to the amount of vegetables. If you have 1 cup of potatoes, add 10 cups of water.

Cover the pot and let it soak for a minimum of 2 hours. If you soak them for longer, change the water about every 3-4 hours.

Once you have allowed them to soak for the time allotted, you should pour out the water and rinse the vegetables again.

Cook the vegetable using a ratio of 5:1 for water to vegetables. Again, if you have 1 cup of potatoes, cook them in 5 cups of water. Eat them.

Other high potassium foods that you can process by leaching are squash, mushrooms, cauliflower, and frozen greens. You should do a slightly different process when leaching those vegetables - follow this process:

Thaw the frozen vegetables to room temperature and drain the excess water.

Rinse the vegetables in warm water. Then fill a pot up - using about 10 times the amount of water to the amount of vegetables.

Cover the pot and let it soak for a minimum of 2 hours. If you soak them for longer, change the water about every 3-4 hours.

Once you have allowed them to soak for the time allotted, you should pour out the water and rinse the vegetables again.

Cook the vegetable using a ratio of 5:1 for water to vegetables. Enjoy them.

I hope that you understand how easy it can be to remove some of the potassium by learning to leach vegetables. This will help you add some variety to your diet without having to eat too many special foods.

What Foods Contain High Amounts Of Potassium?

Potassium is mainly found in certain fruits and vegetables – like bananas, potatoes, avocados, and melons. Potassium can be found in nuts, dried beans, dairy products, and meats. Your body uses potassium for what it needs, and normally it removes the additional potassium with the aid of your kidneys. (There are additional handouts you get that have lists of sodium, potassium, and phosphorus amounts in foods)

Food labels may contain information on how much potassium is in a food, but they are not required to give you that information. They may also tell you the daily value as a percentage for a person. But you might need another source for information on potassium (and phosphorus).

When you are thinking about what to eat – realize how very important the serving size is to the amount of potassium. You can fit many of the high potassium foods in your diet in small amounts. It's really important to realize you will be on this diet for a long time – removing all the potassium from your diet may not be the best option. First of all, you need to eat some! Second of all, you will want it. Making this diet an all or nothing diet is a very short sighted plan. I realize you are scared. It is a reasonable thing to be. You need to get your diet under control. Try some new foods that are low in potassium. You might find that you really like them. However, if you love potatoes, and hate rice, you want to find a way to fit some potatoes into your diet.

Important – Diabetics With A Need To Lower Potassium
If you are a diabetic and you need to treat hypoglycemia, use low potassium foods to affect your blood sugar levels. Use

apple, grape, or cranberry juice to quickly bring up your blood sugars. You may also use glucotabs or jellybeans (about 10) to give you a quick sugar increase. Doing this instead of using orange juice keeps you from taking in too much potassium.

NUTRITION LABEL READING FOR POTASSIUM CONTENT

Food labels are not required to show the amount of potassium per serving. On a label, when you are reading – if it has a daily value for potassium – it is based on 3,500 mg per day. Therefore – if it provides 10% of your daily value for potassium – you have 350 mg of potassium in the serving.

PHOSPHORUS – THE OTHER MINERAL

Now, we get to the 3rd mineral. Once we have figured out where the sodium is and potassium might be, then we realize we must pay attention to one more mineral (maybe). Phosphorus is a mineral that keeps your bones healthy. It keeps your blood vessels and muscles working. Most foods contain some phosphorus (so it's a very limited diet if you want to avoid ALL phosphorus – even the ground contains phosphorus that is absorbed by plants). Aside from just being in most foods, when foods are processed, many times the food processor adds phosphorus.

Needing to manage the protein, sodium, potassium, and now phosphorus is what makes the kidney diet somewhat confusing. If you add diabetes to the mix, you almost lose hope! But don't do that! I'm here to help. Back to our topic, phosphorous.

HOW DO I KNOW IF I SHOULD REDUCE MY PHOSPHORUS INTAKE?

In general, phosphorus intake is naturally reduced when you reduce the amount of protein you eat. As a person with stage 3 or 4 kidney disease, you have already reduced the amount of meat and protein products that you are eating. In many cases, that is enough to control your phosphorus and reduce your risk of further kidney damage.

Your overall goal, and that of your physician, is to maintain your blood phosphorus level within the normal range. Those levels are typically normal until you get into advanced (stage 5 or dialysis) kidney disease. The normal range is: 2.7 – 4.6 mg/dL. If your serum phosphorus (blood level) is elevated, dietary phosphorus restriction should be considered - although the level of restriction is not well researched, it can be best to stay between 800 – 1200 mg per day. If your phosphorus is elevated and you have been instructed to reduce your intake, it would be a good idea to limit your intake of foods with additional phosphate added- read labels for the words "phos" as part of food ingredients.

Why bother at all with phosphorus intake limitations? Controlling phosphorus and calcium levels helps with controlling PTH (Parathyroid Hormone). When you have CKD, your body fails to properly process phosphorus in the kidneys. It then builds up in your blood stream, and pulls potassium or other minerals out of your bones in your body's effort to maintain a balance. This, in turn, makes your bones weak. You might get itchy skin or bone and joint pain. If it's getting too bad, you might need to take a phosphate binder with meals.

Phosphorus binders are often prescribed by your nephrologist to help lower phosphorus levels in your blood by "attaching" to the phosphorus in foods when you eat. That is the reason why you take them when you eat your meals. So, if your doctor has prescribed phosphate binders, you need to take them with meals or they will not be effective. Take your binders within 5-10 minutes of eating both meals and snacks. Take a few less binders with snacks and small meals. This process will help keep your bones healthy. Phosphate binding agents are taken with foods, up to 3-4 times per day, and attach to phosphate in the foods we eat causing it to remain in the digestive system and be excreted through stool. Sometimes doctors use several different types of binders to achieve success. Some phosphate binders can be found over the counter such as calcium carbonate and aluminum hydroxide. But, you should talk to your doctor about it prior to initiating any additional intake.

It is not recommended that people use calcium citrate as a phosphate binder because it can increase your absorption of another mineral – aluminum – that is not desirable. Other binders that your doctor may give you a prescription for are typically composed of resins (sevelamer carbonate) and earth metals (lanthanum carbonate).

WHAT FOODS ARE HIGH OR LOW IN PHOSPHORUS?
Foods that have a lower amount of phosphorus might not be good for you based on your need to lower potassium. You should be aware of all of your restrictions before you start changing your food items that you eat. But you must be aware that if phosphorus is your number one priority – change your foods to be consistent with the biggest priority you have.

Now, onto food items:

I am going to give you guidelines. Foods that are higher in phosphorus are typically meats, poultry, fish, dairy, beans, lentils, nuts, bran cereals and oatmeal, and dark colas. Foods that are lower in phosphorus are fresh fruits and vegetables, rice milk (not enriched), breads, pasta, rice, corn or rice cereals, clear sodas, and home brewed iced tea.

The main thing that you can do to lower phosphorus is to eat a smaller portion of meat. You probably have been doing that because you are on a renal diet. You should eat about 2-3 ounces of meat – about the size of a deck of cards – at a time. You are well on your way to lower phosphorus if you have transitioned to a lower amount of meat.

GENERAL GUIDELINES:
Meats, Poultry and Fish – Limit to a cooked portion of 2-3 ounces per meal

Dairy Foods – Keep your portions of milk or yogurt to ½ cup at a time or one slice of cheese. (Probably around 2-3 servings per day is best) Use non-dairy creamer or rice milk instead of regular milk if you need to use some.

Beans and Lentils – Portions should be about ½ cup of cooked beans or lentils (and replace your meat serving at that meal)

Cola Drinks – You can drink the clear sodas, just not the regular dark colored colas

Chocolate – Limit your intake to occasional treats

Nuts – Keep your portions to about ¼ cup of nuts per day

Fresh Fruits and Vegetables – Mostly ok within boundaries of potassium limitations

Packaged Foods – Look for "phos" on the label. Whole grain cereals can be a big culprit of extra phosphorus

Foods that might have additional phosphorus (added during processing) Frozen uncooked meats and poultry, chicken nuggets, baking mixes, frozen baked goods, cereals, cereal bars, instant puddings and sauces

Additionally, you can change over from whole wheat bread to white bread which is lower in phosphorus as well.

Some foods are important to discuss because they are commonly eaten, and you may find yourself wondering if they are something you need to change. One such example is bread.

WHITE BREAD OR WHOLE WHEAT BREAD ON A KIDNEY DIET? WHICH IS BEST?

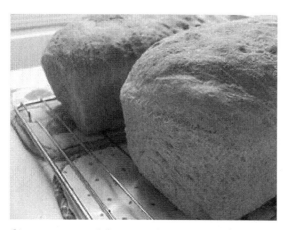

Should I Eat Whole Wheat Bread On A Kidney Diet?

You may have heard not to eat whole wheat bread on a kidney diet, especially on dialysis or as you get closer to stage 5-kidney disease. In addition, these may be foods you once loved. Do you have to give up on wheat bread or not?

WHOLE WHEAT BREAD ON A KIDNEY DIET IS ABOUT POTASSIUM AND PHOSPHORUS

The issues with bread are related to potassium and phosphorus. Foods that are less processed retain much of their potassium and phosphorus naturally. So, the whole grain/ whole wheat bread product has more potassium and phosphorus. It depends on how much you eat and how much potassium and phosphorus your doctor said you should eat in a day. You can eat whole wheat bread without a lot of worry if you manage the rest of your diet with lower amounts of potassium and phosphorus.

DOES IT MATTER HOW MUCH I EAT?

The other thing you should consider is how much of the *whole wheat bread on a kidney diet* that you will be eating. If you eat ½ of a sandwich (1 slice), you won't get as much potassium and phosphorus as you would with 2 slices of bread. So you can eat a smaller portion of bread to allow yourself to eat whole wheat. Otherwise, you should realize you will have to change to eating white bread most of the time – if not all.

The wheat bread that is not **whole wheat bread** is very similar nutritionally to white bread, so if you want to eat bread that is labeled "wheat" and not "whole wheat" you would count it the same as white bread. To be sure it's not whole wheat, make sure it has less than 1 gm of fiber per slice. Whole wheat bread has 1-2 gm of fiber per slice.

WHAT ARE THE SPECIFICS FOR NUTRITIONAL INFORMATION?
Nutritionally, the breakdown of the slices is as follows –
White Bread (.88 oz/slice)
66 calories, 12.7 gm carbohydrate, 0.6 gm fiber, 1.9 gm protein, 170 mg sodium, 25 mg potassium, 25 mg phosphorus
Whole Wheat Bread (1 ounce/slice)
69 calories, 11.6 gm carbohydrate, 1.9 gm fiber, 3.6 gm protein, 132 mg sodium, 69 mg potassium, 57 mg phosphorus

You can see right away that whole wheat bread has more protein, potassium and phosphorus per slice, but less sodium and carbohydrate. But prior to dialysis if your doctor has not recommended a low potassium or low phosphorus diet, you can continue to eat the whole grain wheat breads and get more fiber until you are told differently by your doctor.

I am going to encourage you to **not eliminate all foods with phosphorous** from your diet. You will never get anything to eat as MOST food contains this mineral. Eat smaller portions of these foods that are increased phosphorus and potassium amounts. Take some extra binders. Plan to reduce your intake somewhere else for the day so you can have the items you want.

HOW DOES SECONDARY HYPERPARATHYROIDISM (SHPT) AFFECT MY KIDNEY DISEASE DIET?

Dietary phosphorus restriction and use of active vitamin D (or it's analogs) may help control PTH (parathyroid hormone) levels in CKD. Calcium supplementation may help as well.

First, let me explain what SHPT is. Your parathyroid glands are responsible for keeping your bones and calcium levels in your blood at a healthy range. They are located in your neck on the back of your thyroid gland. Most of the time, you don't even know they are there. They are near your thyroid gland, but work separately and produce PTH (Parathyroid hormone). PTH is responsible for maintaining the correct amount of calcium in the blood and bones, as well as ensuring calcium is absorbed from the digestive system, and finally controlling how much calcium is excreted in the urine. (That is the connection to kidney disease). The amounts of other minerals that are part of bone growth - phosphorus and Vitamin D - are also critically important to the parathyroid. Doctors measure the amount of PTH as an indicator of bone disease.

Secondary Hyperparathyroidism (SHPT) as related to kidney disease is an overproduction of PTH. This is caused by the changes in the kidneys affecting other mineral levels in the blood and causing the body to overproduce PTH. In persons with CKD starting in stage 3, damage to the kidney affects the functioning amount of kidney tissue and cause these changes to start to occur.

WHAT CAUSES THE BODY TO PRODUCE MORE PTH?

While that is a complicated question, I would like to answer it in a way that is easier to understand. Please remember - I am not your doctor!

Initially, your functioning kidney mass is decreased. This happens because of the damage over time to the nephrons in your kidneys. Your doctor may have told you a percentage of your kidneys that are still functioning. Once the amount of your kidneys that are working is decreased beyond a certain level (not exactly clear how much and it varies by individual), 2 things happen.

Calcium regulation

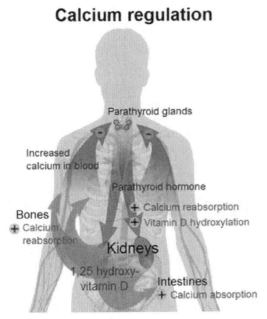

1. Kidneys are responsible to activate the Vitamin D in our body so it works. With less functional kidney, lower amounts of vitamin D3 (active) are available in the blood stream.

2. Kidneys also excrete the phosphorus in our bodies, and with a lower capacity to produce urine, phosphorus builds up in the blood stream.

Those two events that happen over time and bring about a decrease in serum (blood level) calcium. When coupled with a decrease in the amount of Vitamin D3 and an increase in the amount of phosphorus in the blood your body starts to think you need more PTH (because it needs to increase the amount of calcium in your blood stream to a normal level). Our bodies are very efficient at maintaining normal levels in our blood streams and compensate well.

WHAT DOES VITAMIN D DO IN OUR BODY?

PTH works to "normalize" the amount of calcium available in your bloodstream. Calcium is used for many things in your body, and it needs to be available to your cells. So, an increased amount of PTH will cause your bones to be broken down more quickly so that the calcium is available in your bloodstream.

Vitamin D3 happens to be very important in the actions and levels of PTH in our body. You may be aware that our bodies can "make" vitamin D by exposing our skin to sunlight for 10-20 minutes every day. That vitamin D our skin makes has to be transported to the kidney to be changed into the "active" form our body uses. It keeps us from overdosing on Vitamin D with too much sunlight. But you can also get Vitamin D from supplements and milk products that are fortified.

Once vitamin D becomes activated, it can work in our bodies. It stimulates some other hormones that tell the parathyroid we have enough PTH. It also decreases PTH indirectly by increasing the amount of calcium we absorb in our "gut" through our intestines. This increases the amount of calcium in our blood stream, and keeps the amount of PTH at a normal level. But once you have a decreased level of vitamin D in your body, it does not work to increase the level of calcium in your blood stream as efficiently (you don't absorb as much) so your body starts increasing the amount of PTH to accommodate your calcium needs.

SO – decreased Vitamin D levels leads to decreased serum calcium levels causing increased parathyroid hormone levels which increase the amount of calcium removed from the bones leading to bone disease.

How Do Our Bodies Handle Phosphorus?

When the eGFR decreases to less than 60 ml/min, your ability to remove phosphorus from your blood via your kidneys becomes altered. The part of your nephrons that are still working compensate by increasing the removal of phosphorus because your blood levels are increased. This helps to maintain normal phosphorus levels in your blood stream.

Once you progress further in kidney disease, your nephrons eventually become unable to excrete enough phosphorus to compensate, and that is when you start to notice hyperphosphatemia. (elevated blood phosphorus). So, as the amount of phosphorus increases in your blood, PTH is secreted to compensate. Calcium can bind with phosphorus (if they are out of balance) in the blood stream and form particles that then are deposited in organs and blood vessels. As phosphorus levels increase, this risk is higher, so your body reacts by breaking down bones and increasing the calcium levels in the blood stream to even out the levels. This causes the bones to be weakened over time, and calcium particles (those bound with phosphorus) to deposit in areas of the body such as the heart. This is one of the long term complications people often experience on dialysis.

WHAT ARE THE GOALS OF TREATING A PATIENT WITH SHPT?

Overall, the goal is to normalize the levels of the hormones and vitamin D so that the body is not breaking down bone to compensate for increased phosphorus levels. Preventing bone disease, called renal osteodystrophy, is the goal of management of the disease. Patients with kidney disease are at a higher risk of cardiovascular disease, and calcium deposited in the heart can cause further problems.

In stage 3, it is very possible that the levels will be normal, but your body is working overtime to compensate and ensure that you are kept in that normal range. National KDOQI (Kidney Disease Outcomes Quality Initiatives) guidelines recommend that all patients with an eGFR < 60 ml/min/1.73m2 undergo an evaluation of serum calcium, phosphorus and PTH levels. KDOQI guidelines recommend testing once per year starting with the onset of Stage 3 CKD. PTH should be the key test for patients because of the way the body adjusts to keep calcium, Vitamin D, and phosphorus levels in the normal range by increasing the levels of PTH.

Management And Treatment of PTH and SHPT

KDOQI guidelines have recommended target ranges for PTH and calcium levels in patients with Stage 3 - 5 kidney disease. Based on those target ranges, the first course of action to improve the health of a patient with SHPT and suppress the levels of PTH is thought to be Vitamin D therapy. As vitamin D plays such a role in our absorption of calcium, if a person can take in and absorb appropriate amounts of "active" vitamin D (doesn't have to be processed by the kidneys), their calcium absorption rate should also improve. Of course you need to discuss this with your doctor prior to making any sort of changes to your medications.

In addition to Vitamin D, dietary therapy includes reduction of high phosphate foods. Foods that are high in phosphate content include dairy products, meats, beans, dark sodas, beer and nuts. Many of these foods are great sources of protein, so it is important to be cautious when eliminating foods. You should focus on removing foods that are high in phosphate yet lower in protein, such as dark colas, cheese, milk, ice cream and beer.

You have to be careful about sources and amounts of protein because that can lead to malnutrition which affects outcomes once people start on dialysis. Also, dietary phosphate restriction may not be adequate since most of our food contains phosphates. Many doctors also recommend the use of phosphate binders as well.

What Should I Do About SHPT?

First of all, discuss what it means with your doctor. Develop that relationship so you can ask. If you cannot, consider finding another doctor who will work with you. If you need to make a longer appointment, you should tell the person booking the appointment that you have a lot of questions and request a longer appointment time. That will keep your physician from feeling rushed.

At this point - if you have CKD Stage 3, it is recommended that you work with a nephrologist. A nephrologist will follow those KDOQI guidelines to improve your kidney failure and possibly slow the progression of kidney disease. They are experts and will manage your kidney disease very well. Decreasing the amount of phosphate in your diet, in addition to treatment with an active vitamin D medication can provide a great deal of improvement and reduce your risk of bone and cardiac complications.

NUTRITION LABEL READING FOR PHOSPHORUS CONTENT

Food labels are not required to show the amount of phosphorus per serving. On a label, when you are reading – if it has a daily value for phosphorus – it is based on 1,000 mg per day. So – if it provides 10% of your daily value for potassium – you have 100 mg of potassium in the serving.

Remember to read labels and ingredient listings for phosphorus. You can see it identified in the ingredients either as phosphorus or polyphosphates. Avoid processed foods to reduce your intake of phosphorus. Phosphorus is used extensively in processed meats, fish, chicken, leavening agents, and in some powdered drink mixes. Any meat that says it has been "enhanced" is likely high in phosphorus.

Do I Need To Limit My Fluid Intake?

Probably not, unless your Dr. told you that you're on a fluid restriction for your pre-dialysis kidney disease. This usually happens in the later stages of end-stage renal disease, especially when your kidneys are not working to their full capacity. As you lose the ability to urinate, your body retains fluid and increases your blood pressure.

A *fluid restriction* means that you are limited in the amount of fluid or products that become fluid at room temperature that you can take in because your body is not removing the fluid properly.

If you have too much fluid in your body and it's not removed in a timely manner, it can aggravate high blood pressure, it can cause fluid in the lungs, and it can cause other problems with your heart. Complications from extra fluid also involves swollen legs, and fatigue. Your fluid restriction amount would be determined specifically by your doctors, but ask them for specifics such as how many ounces or milliliters you are allowed. Fluid restrictions are to make the patient feel more comfortable and reduce the weight gain that you have. Because if you take in fluids and you can't get rid of them, the water just stays on your body as weight and can make you very uncomfortable. This may be referred to as edema by your nurses or doctors.

What Is A Fluid on A Kidney Diet For A Fluid Restriction?

While it's obvious that beverages like water, coffee, juice, soda and other liquids or shakes count as fluid, other food items may not be as obvious. Ice, ice cream and sherbet, gelatin, popsicles, and soup also count as fluid amount since they become liquid at room temperature or body temperature when they enter your stomach. Fruits and some vegetables also contain liquid, and you may want to check specifically with your doctor if you need to monitor your fluid intake closely for those items. But in general, anything that is liquid at room temperature counts as a fluid.

Fruits and vegetables they generally don't count as part of your fluid allowance but do contain a significant amount of fluid are: apples, blueberries, blackberries, broccoli, cabbage, cauliflower, carrots, celery, cherries, cranberries, cucumbers, eggplant, grapes, lettuce, peaches, pears, peppers, pineapple, plums, strawberries, tangerines, and zucchini.

GOOD WAYS TO LIMIT YOUR FLUID ON A FLUID RESTRICTION
- While your fluid needs will depend on your weight and height, and be directed to you specifically by your nephrologist or doctor, some ideas on how to limit and inyour fluid intake might be helpful.
- Don't do things that increase your thirst such as eating salty or spicy foods. Overall you should reduce your salt intake not only for your kidney diet but also to keep you from increasing your thirst.
- Spread your liquids out throughout the day don't drink all of them in the morning and then have nothing left for your evening meal.
- Don't get overheated by exercising or being outside in the heat, stay in the cool areas.
- Use smaller cups as they make you feel like you're getting a bigger amount without noticing that it's really a limited portion.
- Try making ice cubes out of your favorite beverage, and then when you're thirsty you can chew on those ice cubes as part of your daily limit but they will last a little longer because they're cold and they take a while longer to melt.
- It's really important to keep a daily fluid and food journal including your way information. If your doctors have put you on a fluid restriction that means they are concerned about the amount of fluid that you

may be taking in and not being able to process through your kidneys. Keeping a journal will help you to understand where your problems may have occurred and discuss them with your doctors.

MEAL PLANNER TRACKING GUIDE

Use the meal planning guide on the next page to track your meals. We have also included several pages of information on the amount of potassium and phosphorus in some common foods. Since the amount of protein and sodium is already located on the label, we felt that if those are the only two nutrients you need to be concerned with, then don't complicate it. (It's complicated enough). If you do need to track, you will want to choose based on your ability to eat either potassium or phosphorus if your physician has given you a restriction. (Many times people think they need to be on a potassium restriction, and they just really need to eat less protein and sodium and it will improve their kidneys).

You can get this meal planner in a full size form via email. Sign up and learn more about specific foods you can eat more or less of.

Go to: http://www.renaldiethq.com/book2files/

Meal	Protein	Sodium	Potassium	Phosphorus	Fluid
Breakfast					
Lunch					
Dinner					
Snacks					
Total for Day					
Recommended Amt	_____ g	_____ mg	_____ mg	_____ mg	_____ oz

CHART OF POTASSIUM AND PHOSPHOROUS FOOD VALUES

These are available through the email signup which is free and used to provide the files. You will find two different lists – one sorted by type of food – beverage, fruit, juice, etc. And one sorted with the lowest potassium foods at the beginning, just in case you are looking for something low in potassium to eat. Each list is the exact same, just sorted differently. They are 11 pages each.

Go to: http://www.renaldiethq.com/book2files/

Next Steps

1. Eating less protein will help your kidneys most of all because it means you will naturally reduce the amounts of nutrients you need.

2. Start tracking your sodium intake. Everyone needs to limit their sodium, including those with just stage 1 or 2 kidney disease. Use the guides, or make your own, but start writing down the amount of protein and sodium you eat. Do that for at least a week.

3. Once you are able to get your sodium intake down to about 1500 mg/day, IF you need to limit your potassium and phosphorus, please start tracking those as well. You should know based on your labs and information from your doctors if you need to limit your potassium or phosphorus. If you don't – yeah, one less restriction. If you do, keep track of the amount of potassium and phosphorus in all the food you eat using the charts provided.

4. Strive for variety in all things that you do. Do not limit your meals so severely that you can only eat one meal. You will quickly become bored and give up. And my hope for you is that you can implement this info and see an improvement in your outcomes. Use the guides provided, via email, to find good foods you can eat. And remember that you can have some of the higher potassium and phosphorus foods – just in limited amounts.

5. Know your labs – where you started and where you are going (your sodium, phosphorous and potassium numbers). You need that guidepost to understand your own situation. Talk to your doctor about anything that seems out of whack and how you can fix it. Ask before starting any new over the counter medication or supplements.

Don't forget to get the potassium and phosphorus lists – Go to: http://www.renaldiethq.com/book2files/

They are FREE and you do not have to purchase them. If you have difficulty getting to the files, let me know at **contact@renaldiethq.com**

I want you to be satisfied. Please contact me with any issues.

CONGRATULATIONS! KEEP UP THE GOOD WORK, YOU ARE ON YOUR WAY TO A HEALTHIER YOU!

About Me

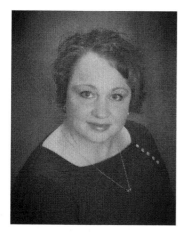

Thank you so much for your support and purchase of this book! I hope you will give it an honest review, that helps others decide if it's the right book for them.

I want to remind you about the free E-course that is part of this book – added information about related topics that you can use to improve your cooking and health.

Go to: http://www.renaldiethq.com/go/book2notify

A little bit about me, I am a registered dietitian nutritionist in Oklahoma. I have been working in the field since 1996. I have an MBA and I love to cook. I am married and have 2 children. I work as an adjunct professor locally at one of the colleges, teaching food service management. I understand making menus and how to create recipes that are healthy and tasty. As a dietitian for so long, I have spoken with many of you who struggle with chronic kidney disease, and I want to help. You can always find more information and articles at my website dedicated to that topic at: http://www.renaldiethq.com/

I also have a podcast on iTunes at:
http://www.renaldiethq.com/go/itunes

I have a YouTube channel where I often do live events talking about renal and kidney disease:
http://www.youtube.com/RenalDietHQ

I would love to have you in the Face book group:
http://www.renaldiethq.com/facebookgroup

I also have a Google+ group if you prefer:
http://www.renaldiethq.com/talkingkidneydisease

Find Us On Pinterest:
http://www.pinterest.com/matheaford/

Find Us On Twitter: https://twitter.com/RenalDietHQ

OTHER TITLES BY MATHEA FORD:

Mathea Ford, Author Page (all books):

http://www.amazon.com/Mathea-Ford/e/B008E1E7IS/

The Kidney Friendly Diet Cookbook

http://www.amazon.com/Kidney-Friendly-Diet-Cookbook-PreDialysis-ebook/dp/B00BC7BGPI/

Create Your Own Kidney Diet Plan

http://www.amazon.com/Create-Your-Kidney-Diet-Plan-ebook/dp/B009PSN3R0/

Living with Chronic Kidney Disease - Pre-Dialysis

http://www.amazon.com/Living-Chronic-Kidney-Disease-Pre-Dialysis-ebook/dp/B008D8RSAQ/

Eating a Pre-Dialysis Kidney Diet - Calories, Carbohydrates, Fat & Protein, Secrets To Avoid Dialysis

http://www.amazon.com/Eating-Pre-Dialysis-Kidney-Diet-Carbohydrates-ebook/dp/B00DU2JCHM/

Eating a Pre-Dialysis Kidney Diet - Sodium, Potassium, Phosphorus and Fluids, A Kidney Disease Solution

http://www.amazon.com/Eating-Pre-Dialysis-Kidney-Diet-Phosphorus-ebook/dp/B00E2U8VMS/

Eating Out On a Kidney Diet: Pre-dialysis and Diabetes: Ways To Enjoy Your Favorite Foods

http://www.amazon.com/Eating-Out-Kidney-Diet-Pre-dialysis/dp/0615928781/

Kidney Disease: Common Labs and Medical Terminology: The Patient's Perspective

http://www.amazon.com/Kidney-Disease-Terminology-Perspective-Pre-Dialysis/dp/0615931804/

Dialysis: Treatment Options for the Progression to End Stage Renal Disease

http://www.amazon.com/Dialysis-Treatment-Options-Progression-Disease/dp/0615932258/

Mindful Eating For A Pre-Dialysis Kidney Diet: Healthy Attitudes Toward Food and Life

http://www.amazon.com/Mindful-Eating-Pre-Dialysis-Kidney-Diet/dp/0615933475/

The Emotional Challenges Of Coping with Chronic Kidney Disease

http://www.amazon.com/Emotional-Challenges-Chronic-Disease-Dialysis-ebook/dp/B00H6SYQG8/

Heart Healthy Living with Kidney Disease: Lowering Blood Pressure

http://www.amazon.com/Heart-Healthy-Living-Kidney-Disease/dp/0615936059/

Exercising with Chronic Kidney Disease: Solutions To An Active Lifestyle http://www.amazon.com/Exercising-Chronic-Kidney-Disease-Solutions/dp/0615936342/

Sexuality and Chronic Kidney Disease For Men and Women: A Path To Better Understanding

http://www.amazon.com/Sexuality-Chronic-Kidney-Disease-Women/dp/0615960197/

Anemia and Chronic Kidney Disease: Signs, Symptoms, and Treatment for Anemia in Kidney Failure

http://www.amazon.com/Anemia-Chronic-Kidney-Disease-Treatment/dp/0692201416/

Alternative Treatment Options For Chronic Kidney Failure: Natural Remedies for Living a Healthier Life

http://www.amazon.com/Alternative-Treatment-Options-Chronic-Failure/dp/0692281916/

Caring for Renal Patients: A guide to taking care of your loved ones who are struggling with kidney failure

http://www.amazon.com/Headquarters-Disease-Patients-Educational-Worksheets/dp/B00LZ2ICPW/

Positive Beginnings: The Dialysis Breakfast Cookbook

http://www.amazon.com/Positive-Beginnings-Dialysis-Breakfast-Cookbook/dp/069227958X/

Sign up for our email list to learn of new titles right away!

http://www.renaldiethq.com/go/email/

Made in the USA
San Bernardino, CA
11 May 2019